Candida Cleanse

Cure Candida & Restore Your Health in 21 Days

Christine Weil

Table of Contents

Introduction

I want to thank you and congratulate you for purchasing, *"Candida Cleanse: Cure Candida and Restore Your Health Naturally in 21 days"*.

This book contains proven steps and strategies to treat and prevent Candida in 21 days, starting from diagnosis, to colonic irrigations, the diet, sustained healing and preventing a reoccurrence.

The one thing we need to accept is the fact that fungi are everywhere; these small single celled organisms can be found in land, water and the air. It is estimated there is over 500,000 species of fungi on our planet; recently more attention is being given to the common fungi called Candida. Not only are they part of our digestive system, but our lifestyle can cause an overgrowth of Candida, which can be difficult to heal, once it in our bloodstream. This guide will show you how to treat, heal and prevent an overgrowth.

Thanks again for purchasing this book, I hope you enjoy it!

Christine Weil

What is Candida Albicans?

What is Candida Albicans?

Candida yeast is a type of fungus, a microorganism that is not beneficial for the body; which is why it is referred to as "unfriendly" bacteria. It exists everywhere and humans can come into contract with it throughout their normal day. Candida is on everything you touch, the air you breathe and on most of the food you consume. While it usually isn't a problem, if it becomes overgrown, the fungus interferes with the friendly bacteria in the body. This overgrowth of Candida leads to all kinds of health problems.

Who can Contract It?

Candida can effect men, women, and children-even though it is thought to be an infection only women encounter through yeast infections. The main habitat for this yeast is the digestive tract. This yeast can manifest itself in many forms, such as dandruff, white flaky skin, vaginal discharge, jock itch, athlete's foot, white coating on the tongue in adults, colic and thrush in children.

As many as 90% or more North Americans may be suffering the effects of Candida and not realize what it is. The side effects of a yeast overgrowth can result in: allergies, anxiety, asthma, acne, bloating, chemical sensitivities, coughs, cramps, constipation, chronic fatigue syndrome, trouble concentrating, diarrhea, eczema, fuzzy thinking, gas, gastritis, headaches, hives, hyperactivity, migraines, sore throats, rashes, nausea, sinus pressure, thrush and vaginal yeast infections

If you believe or know you have an overgrowth of yeast, this book will provide guidelines for diagnosing, understanding

and treating it with natural remedies, prescription drugs, wholesome foods and recipes and lifestyle changes.
Moderate cases of yeast infestations can be healed within a 21 day period, which includes the Candida Cleanse and Colonic irrigation.

The more serious or stubborn cases of yeast can take as long as 6 to 12 months, depending upon the methods used to heal the problem. It can recur, which makes it difficult to fully cure, you have to continue practicing prevention methods and make permanent changes in your lifestyle to completely heal and clean the body of the overabundance of the yeast.

To cure Candida, it is necessary to destroy as much of the yeast as possible and restore a healthful balance of friendly bacteria within the body. The overgrowth must be kept under control by consuming foods and water that do not feed on the yeast. Because it is the body's natural defense system that keeps the overgrowth in check we have to increase and then maintain the body's energy levels to keep the yeast from regaining control.

How Do You Know if You Have Candida?

This yeast infection is difficult to diagnose, and the medical profession is skeptical that it can be an underlying cause of many ailments, and one of the mysteries concerning Candida is that, when tested for, it can give false positive and negative results. There are many questionnaires available, but these can over or under diagnose the problem.

The symptoms of the overgrowth can resemble other illnesses, such as allergies, rashes, cold like symptoms, etc. So what are the most common symptoms of over growth?

Common Symptoms:

1. **General:** Chronic fatigue, sugar and bread cravings, reactions to perfumes, tobacco, chemicals, craving for alcoholic beverages

2. **Gastrointestinal:** Thrush, bloating, gas, intestinal cramps, rectal itching, alternating diarrhea and constipation.

3. **Genitourinary system:** Vaginal yeast infections, frequent bladder infections, bloating, fluid retention, cramps, genital rashes, persistent prostatis.

4. **Hormonal system:** Menstrual irregularities, decreased libido, hypothyroidism, hyperthyroidism.

5. **Nervous system:** Depression, irritability, trouble concentrating, feeling spacey, anxiety, memory loss, insomnia, mood swings, numbness, tingling of extremities.

6. **Immune system:** Allergies, lowered resistance to infections.

7. **Skin:** chronic rashes, itching, psoriasis, recurrent hives, ringworm, athlete's foot, chronic fungal nail or skin infections, foot, hair and body odors not relieved by washing.

When these organisms are allowed to grow the balance between yeast and bacteria become upset resulting in *intestinal candidiasis* – also called the yeast syndrome.

When the yeast dies it releases protein fragments and toxins; which can be absorbed into the bloodstream and then travel to many areas of the body. The immune system attempts to deal with these toxins causing a variety of symptoms like the ones we just addresses. It can be a main cause of many chronic and difficult to diagnose health conditions.

Factors Which Increase the Risk of Overgrowth

1. Repeated use of antibiotics and/or steroids

2. Chronic stress, anxiety, depression,

3. Diet high in simple sugars

4. Alcohol usage

5. Oral contraceptive use, female hormone replacement therapy

6. Diabetes

7. Hypothyroidism

8. Weakened immune system

Candida and Our Lifestyle

Today many of the foods we have traditionally consider "healthy" have been found to be heavily colonized by fungi and their toxins. These include corn, peanuts, cashews and dried coconut. In a lesser degree fungi can be found in breads of all kinds, barley, rye, wheat white rice, millet and many cereal grains. Candida loves these foods, and use them as a base to colonize in the gastrointestinal tract and increase the risk of overpopulation of the yeast.

Cigarette smoking not only can contribute to lung cancer, because of the carcinogens, but the cigarettes themselves are also contaminated with fungi in the sugar and yeast used to hold them together. The fungal contamination increases their harmful effects on our body, assisting with the growth.

Many of our favorite foods and beverages undergo fungal fermentation such as; bread, wine, beer, cheeses, and aged or cured meats. Small amounts of these products have little effect on people with healthy immune systems, but for those with chronic conditions, they can be deadly.

Candida and its toxins can travel to most of our organs and tissues throughout the body. This yeast syndrome can contribute to the causes of many illnesses such as chronic sinusitis, recurrent flu and colds, middle ear infections, alcoholism, asthma, eating disorders, and many other conditions. A healthy immune system is the best defense against these toxins.

Our Lifestyle Maintains Growth

The things we put into our systems have a great effect on our bodies, so let's elaborate on the major contributing factors to Candida overgrowth:

Antibiotics-We have overused antibiotics; they have been prescribed for every illness, for prevention and even for acne outbreaks. Antibiotics are the most common cause of the overgrowth. Antibiotics destroy our harmful bacteria and our good bacteria. When our friendly bacteria are destroyed it gives the organism a chance to multiply. Anyone who has taken an antibiotic for more than one course for 7-10 days is at risk for yeast infection.

Birth Control Pills- Oral birth control pills are made of estrogen in a synthetic form. This synthetic estrogen has been found to promote Candida overgrowth.

Excessive Stress- Stress can cause the growth, because when we are stressed we release the hormone cortisol. Cortisol can weaken our immune system and raise blood sugar levels. With the rise in blood sugar the yeast can feed on it and allow it to multiply. When we are depressed our immune system is affected and it becomes defenseless against the overgrowth of yeast.

Tap water- Common tap water is high in chlorine which destroys friendly intestinal bacteria giving yeast a nice environment to grow in.

Parasites and Intestinal worms- Researchers have estimated that over 85% of all people in North America have parasites. They can be large worm-like creatures or small microscopic organisms, and they destroy the friendly bacteria in the intestines making overgrowth possible.

Constipation- Candida can be the cause of your constipation, just as constipation can lead to the overgrowth in the first place. When we have constipation our digestive tract becomes more alkaline, which creates the perfect environment for the yeast to grow and multiply.

Alcohol- excessive use of alcohol can destroy the good bacterium thereby allowing an overgrowth of yeast. Because of its maltose content, beer especially can become a real problem. Maltose is a sugar derived from malt and is a potent yeast cell fuel. All alcohol should be used in moderation and not at all when you have been diagnosed with Candida.

How is it Diagnosed?

Yeast, mold and fungi are present everywhere thriving on every surface of all living things. To diagnose Candida your physician will do a complete medical history and ask you to complete a questionnaire which can show the probability of whether you have or don't have overgrowth. A stool sample will be taken and is tested and/or blood test may be ordered. The stool sample is called a Comprehensive Digestive Stool Analysis-which is a group of 25 tests performed on a stool sample which reveal information about your digestive system.

This test can evaluate:

1. Digestion of food molecules and absorption of nutrients.
2. Presences of yeast or bacterial infection.
3. Intestinal flora balance
4. Intestinal immune function

5.   Dietary fiber intake

Treatment is monitored by your physician through the use of antifungal and standard medications.

Standard and Antifungal Medications Prescribed by Physicians

Gastrzyme- This is a source of Vitamin U and other nutrients known to help resolve stomach inflammation and ulcers. Vitamin U is a cabbage extract which is very high in chlorophyll, which kills t yeast. Vitamin U comes in capsule/tablet form and is safe and effective.

ADP- Is a standardized extract of the oil of oregano in an emulsified in a sustained release form. It should be taken just before meals on an empty stomach. ADP is useful in ridding the body of excessive levels of yeast. ADP acts like an antibiotic and actually sterilizes the bowel.

Bio-B100- Is a multiple B vitamin containing the natural forms of B-1, B-2, and B-6 and combines both the B and G factors. Coffee, alcohol, tobacco, sugar, estrogen therapy and birth control pills interfere with B vitamin absorption causing a greater need for them to prevent growth.

There are many other medications and treatments available, too many to cover in this guide. Your physician and you together will decide on the right course of treatment for you, determining the severity of your overgrowth.

Additional Recommendations

- Are you a coffee drinker? Coffee can kill up to 75% of the friendly flora in the colon per cup, and decaffeinated coffee is just as bad. It takes the body 5 hours to replace the flora lost from a single cup of Joe!

- Avoid using antibiotics and steroids unless it is absolutely necessary.

- Follow the Candida Diet (more on that in a bit).

- Stop using birth control pills. The progesterone of these pills causes changes in the vaginal mucus membrane which makes it easier for Candida to multiply.

Natural Candida Treatments

Natural Remedies for Candida

Acidophilus- The beneficial bacteria acidophilus is thought to control Candida by making the intestinal tract more acidic, discouraging the growth of Candida and by producing hydrogen peroxide which directly kills Candida. Research has shown that supplementing with a hydrogen peroxide producing strain of acidophilus (DDS-1) greatly reduced the incidence of antibiotic induced yeast infections. These beneficial bacteria also help to restore the microbial balance within the digestive tract.

Warning: this is hydrogen peroxide manufactured from the complex processes in our bodies, not the hydrogen peroxide you can purchase in a store. **DO NOT** consume hydrogen peroxide!

Fiber- One teaspoon to one tablespoon of soluble fiber containing guar gum, psylluim husks, flaxseed or pectin can be mixed in an 8 ounce glass of water two times per day on an empty stomach. Fiber assists in pushing the waste products and yeast out of our gastrointestinal tract.

Enteric coated essential oils- Enteric coated capsules containing oregano oil, peppermint oil and other volatile oils are believed to prevent the overgrowth. It is usually recommended for at least several months. A standard dosage is 2 capsules 2 times daily with water in between meals. Pure essential oils can be quite toxic in this amount, so the liquid form of these oils should never be ingested and the capsules should not be broken open before ingesting.

Enteric coated garlic- Garlic capsules that have been enteric coated are made this way so they open when they reach the intestines, are often used in combination with the essential oils. One capsule two time per day taken with the enteric coated essential oils is a standard recommendation. Other valuable supplements are Caprylic acid from coconuts, oleic oil from olive oil, oregano oil and Pau d'arco.

Diet- Diet is an important part of the Cleanse. The length of time on the Cleanse depends on the length of time one has had symptoms, the symptom severity and overall health. People may notice improvement after strict adherence to the diet for 2 to 3 weeks. For others it may take as long as several months. Once symptoms are gone and lab tests show significant improvement, foods from the restricted list can be slowly incorporated back into the diet.

Natural Antifungal Antifungals are natural alternative products which can be obtained from a health food store and some drug stores. They assist in the prevention and treatment of yeast infections by killing the yeast and cleansing the colon. The following antifungals are effective and recommended treatments by holistic practitioners (if you have a health condition, talk to your physician before you try these alternative medicines.)

1. Aloe Vera
2. Black Walnut
3. Caprylic Acid
4. Cloves
5. Garlic
6. Goldenseal
7. Grapefruit Seed
8. Olive Oil Extract
9. Oregano Oil
10. Pau d'Arco

Aloe Vera

Aloe is great for general intestinal health. It contains enzymes that help break down fats, sugars, and starches, and promotes the growth of healthy bacteria in the intestine. The yeast breeds in your intestine when passage time is too long, but Aloe can help by alleviating constipation.

The colon is another point in your body where toxins collect, and Aloe's mild laxative effect loosens the toxin buildup and flushes it though your system. In addition, Aloe Vera repairs and heals your intestinal wall, which stops the yeast from actually flushing through into your blood stream.

Aloe Vera is a great detoxifier for the entire body, but especially for the overburdened liver – the organ that cleans the toxins from your blood.

How do you take Aloe Vera?

Aloe Vera juice can be found at any health food store. If you don't like the taste, you can add a squeeze of lemon. It also comes in a concentrated capsule form. Dosage should be no more than a quarter of a cup a day. You can start with half the dose to make sure it doesn't cause any stomach cramps.

Aloe Vera Side Effects?

Extended use of Aloe Vera can cause allergies such as hives or rash with some people.

Black Walnut

In a scientific study, Black Walnut husks were shown to combat the yeast better than several commercial antifungal drugs. Black Walnut is now found in many over the counter cures, but is also available in concentrated form.

The bark, husk and leaves of the Black Walnut tree have been used as medicine for centuries in North America – the bark for toothache, the inner bark as a laxative, the juice for ringworm and the leaves for bedbugs and mites.

How does Black Walnut work?

"In a 1990 University of Mississippi study the active ingredient in black walnut called juglone, was shown to be as effective as some commercial antifungal. According to the study, the test results "for juglone showed it to have moderate antifungal activity and to be as effective as certain commercially available antifungal agents such as zinc undecylenate and selenium sulfide."

Black Walnut contains natural tannins that kill parasites, yeast and fungus. Juglone has some antibiotic and antifungal effects.

Other benefits of Black Walnut are in attacking worms and yeast infections. It may also help with lowering blood pressure, thyroid problems, diarrhea, sore throats and asthma.

How do you take Black Walnut?

The best form of Black Walnut to take is the husk (or hull). The nut is harvested when green and then soaked to remove the husk. It is then soaked and the extract removed. It is as an extract that Black Walnut is most effective.

Black Walnut extract is usually sold as a tincture, or alcoholic solution. Don't worry about the alcoholic effect – it is used in such small quantities that this effect is minimal.

Who should not take Black Walnut?

Those who have existing liver or kidney conditions should be careful with Black Walnut as it may irritate these organs. Pregnant or breastfeeding women should also avoid taking it, as should those with gastrointestinal conditions.

Black Walnut Side Effects?

No side effects have been reported in humans taking Black Walnut. It does however contain high levels of *tannins*, chemicals that have previously been linked with damage to the liver and kidneys, so care should be taken and consult with your medical professional before taking Black Walnut.

Caprylic Acid

Caprylic Acid is a naturally occurring antifungal fatty acid that is found in coconut oil. It is a potent antifungal that kills yeast cells, as well as restoring your stomach acidity to its normal levels. You can start taking caprylic acid as soon as you have finished your cleanse in the first stage of the diet. It is available in gel capsules, which allow the caprylic acid to get to your intestinal tract and start killing Candida cells.

Natural antifungals like caprylic acid work best in combination, as this prevents the yeast from adapting to a single treatment. So you can combine caprylic acid with other natural antifungals like oregano oil, garlic and grapefruit seed extract. Caprylic acid works primarily in the gastrointestinal tract, killing the bad cells.

How does Caprylic Acid help with an overgrowth?

Like other antifungals, caprylic acid works by interfering with the cell walls of the yeast. Repeated studies have shown its effectiveness against Candida.

According to a study conducted by Japan's Niigata University, *"the fungicidal effect of caprylic acid on Candida Albicans was exceedingly powerful"*. You can begin taking antifungals like caprylic acid as soon as you have finished your cleanse in the first stage of the diet.

Caprylic acid also helps to normalize the acidity in your stomach. Stomach acidity is important because it allows your immune system to function properly, enabling it to fight off the overgrowth. Caprylic Acid helps to restore a natural, acidic environment to your stomach.

How do you take Caprylic Acid?

You can buy Caprylic Acid in capsules. You should take these capsules with meals, twice daily. These gel capsules are for the most part are effective because they slow the release of the caprylic acid, allowing its antifungal properties to take effect in your intestinal tract.

Coconut oil contains caprylic acid, lauric acid and capric acid, three potent antifungals that work great in combination. You can start with 1-2 tablespoons of coconut oil each morning, then build up your dosage to 5 tablespoons per day if you don't experience any Die-Off symptoms.

Who should not take Caprylic Acid?

Pregnant or breastfeeding women, children and those prone to stomach upsets should not take Caprylic Acid. Caprylic acid may sometimes cause mild gastrointestinal complaints, like nausea or diarrhea. If you are in any doubt, consult your doctor.

Cloves

Cloves come from the evergreen clove tree, common in Indonesia but now found around the world.

How do Cloves work?

Along with their other medical benefits, cloves are also a powerful anti-fungal agent often used to treat athletes foot and other fungal infections Its antiseptic properties allow it to kill the Candida yeast, while it also boosts your immune system.

Clove extract is most effective in the oil form. Add 15 to 30 drops in warm water and take this tea 1-3 times daily. Be sure to dilute it; clove extract is actually quite a powerful substance.

Clove oil also blends quite well with other essential oils, such as basil essential oil, rosemary essential oil, rose oil, cinnamon essential oil and grapefruit essential oil.

Who shouldn't take Cloves?

Check with your doctor regarding the use of clove oil during pregnancy or breastfeeding. Also take advice if you are seriously ill, especially with a gastrointestinal problem. Some people may have an allergic reaction to cloves so start with a small dose.

Clove Side Effects

Cloves are a powerful spice and should never be taken in large quantities. If taken in too great a quantity, especially in undiluted oil, the following side effects may be experienced:

1. Vomiting
2. Sore Throat

3. Seizure
4. Sedation
5. Difficulty breathing
6. Hematemesis
7. Kidney Failure
8. Liver damage
9. Erectile dysfunction
10. Problems with ejaculation
11. Seizure
12. Stomach irritation

If you are careful with your dosage and start small, you should have no problems with cloves or clove oil.

Garlic

Garlic is a proven antifungal that is a simple and easy addition to your treatment plan. Research studies have shown that garlic is effective against these pathogens. In addition to its use as an antifungal garlic can support your immune system, reduce cholesterol, and help control blood sugar levels.

You can start taking garlic supplements once you have finished your cleanse and moved on to the strict Candida diet. As always, it is better to take two or three antifungals at once to prevent the yeast from adapting, so you can use garlic in addition to other natural antifungals.

How does Garlic help with overgrowth?

There is a wide range of scientific research and information supporting the use of garlic as an antifungal. One of the key compounds in garlic is *ajoene*, a proven antifungal that has been shown to be effective against many fungal strains. *Ajoene* is formed from a compound named *allicin* and an enzyme named *allinase*. When these two natural compounds come into contact (by chopping the garlic, crushing it or by other means), they form an antibacterial agent named allicin, which then combines to form *ajoene.*

Although this has proven antifungal properties, the exact method by which this happens is not clear. As with other antifungals, scientists suspect that it works by disturbing the cells walls of the yeast cells.

A major benefit of garlic is that it is so easy to include in your treatment plan. Garlic tablets, softgels and oils are widely available, and fresh garlic cloves make a tasty addition to many recipes. You can use garlic as an accompaniment to your other antifungals without having to spend a great deal of money. To get the best results and prevent the yeast from adapting to the treatment, it is best to take two or three antifungals at the same time.

How do you take Garlic?

Garlic products can be found in a number of different forms, in both your supermarket and your health food store. In your supermarket you will find items like fresh garlic cloves, garlic paste, crushed garlic, garlic flakes or garlic powder. Your health food store should stock garlic tablets and garlic oil.

Each type contains different levels of the active ingredients, so make sure to read the ingredients and take as directed.

Who should not take Garlic?

Although a natural remedy, concentrated garlic can still interact with other medicines, so always consult a health professional. Garlic has a blood-thinning property that can be very useful, but can also be dangerous to sufferers of hemophilia or platelet disorders, as well as pregnant women or patients about to undergo surgery.

Side effects from garlic include upset stomach, bloating, bad breath, body odor, and a stinging sensation on the skin from handling too much fresh or dried garlic. Handling garlic may also cause the appearance of skin lesions.

Other side effects that have been reported by those taking garlic supplements include headache, fatigue, loss of appetite, muscle aches, dizziness described as vertigo (namely, the room spinning), and allergies such as an asthmatic reaction or contact dermatitis (skin rash).

Some people may suffer a mild allergic reaction to concentrated garlic. Others may have an upset stomach, body odor, bad breath, headache, loss of appetite or fatigue. It may prompt a skin reaction, such as a stinging in the hands.

Goldenseal

Goldenseal was originally used for skin disorders, digestive complaints and even as a cancer remedy. In more modern times, Goldenseal has gained in popularity and has been used for wound healing and many types of infection, as well as an antifungal agent for ailments like yeast overgrowth. Goldenseal helps heal fungal infections by encouraging the growth of friendly intestinal bacteria and is a valuable supplement to help prevent the growth.

You can start taking antifungals like goldenseal soon after you complete the cleanse and move on to the diet. If you combine goldenseal with other antifungals, you will reduce the chance of it adapting to the treatment.

How does Goldenseal help with a Candida overgrowth?

The active ingredient in goldenseal is *berberine*, an alkaloid that is also found in other plants such as barberry. *Berberine* inhibits the growth of various species. *Berberine* has been shown to help regulate blood sugar levels, preventing the spikes that can feed a overgrowth.

Berberine helps with the infestations in another way too. It activates the white blood cells in your body, thereby strengthening your immune system and enhancing your body's ability to fight off infections by itself.

How do you take Goldenseal?

Goldenseal is generally sold either as a liquid extract of the goldenseal root, or as capsules made from goldenseal root powder. If you buy the liquid form, you will need to take a few drops in water, 1-3 times a day, and the bottle will often come with a dropper to measure the exact amount. The capsules are also taken several times a day, and dosage will depend on the strength of the preparation. Be sure to follow the instructions on the bottle.
Also be careful not to take too much Goldenseal, as large quantities can irritate the liver. It's better to start with a small dose (below the manufacturer's recommended amount), then slowly increase it. You can take goldenseal in combination with other natural antifungal remedies, to prevent the yeast from adapting to a single antifungal.

Who should not take Goldenseal?

Those who are pregnant or breastfeeding should not take goldenseal. A major ingredient, Berberine, can caused uterine contractions and may cause problems with the pregnancy. Those with kidney disease, liver disease, heart disease, or other serious conditions should consult with their doctor first.

Many users report a feeling of nervousness when taking goldenseal. Others report irritations in their throat and occasionally digestive problems.

Grapefruit Seed Extract

Although grapefruit seed extract was not widely used until the 1970s, its use since then has increased as both doctors and patients have realized its broad applications against all kinds of infections, including overgrowth.

Grapefruit seed extract has been found to perform as well or better than 30 antibiotics and 18 fungicides. However, as a non-toxic, natural remedy, it had none of the side effects of the other treatments!

Grapefruit seed extract has a great selection of vitamins that can both do wonders for your general health, and also help you through your treatment for yeast infestation. It boosts your immune system and helps to repair liver cells that may be damaged by the release of toxins in a Die-Off reaction.

How does Grapefruit Seed Extract help with Candida overgrowth?

Grapefruit seed also has a number of important chemicals – Vitamins C & E, bioflavonoids – that can help repair cells in the body. One particular bioflavanoid, named *Hesperedin*, can give a natural boost to your immune system. The natural acidity of the extract also helps your immune system by restoring your stomach to its natural pH (it can frequently become too alkaline during an overgrowth).

The great thing about taking grapefruit seed extract for digestive complaints is that it leaves the beneficial bacteria in your system intact. Compare that to other antimicrobial treatments that can leave your intestine empty of these helpful organisms.

What is Grapefruit Seed Extract?

Grapefruit Extract is made by mixing grapefruit seeds and pulp into a thick, highly acidic liquid. After some further processing, you are left with a yellow, viscous liquid that has a strong bitter taste. It is usually mixed with vegetable glycerin to reduce the bitterness and acidity.

Grapefruit seed extract is sold either as a liquid concentrate or in tablets. Both contain the vegetable glycerin, but the tablets will also contain a small amount of filler, such as organic brown rice protein. This is OK in small amounts on a Candida diet.

How do you take Grapefruit Seed Extract?

The extract usually comes in liquid concentrate or tablet form. If taking the liquid concentrate, 10 drops in a cup of water is a typical dose, to be taken 3 times a day. In tablet form, 100-200mg three times a day should be sufficient. Always read the label and follow the manufacturer's instructions.

Who should not take Grapefruit Seed Extract?

As always, users with serious health conditions should consult their doctor before taking it. Grapefruit seed extract does interact with a number of common medicines so do keep this in mind and inform your doctor of all medications that you are taking.

Olive Leaf Extract

Derivative from the leaves of the olive tree, Olive Leaf Extract contains an active ingredient named *Oleuropein*, which is showing positive results in numerous studies as a yeast killer.

This powerful herbal remedy is a natural and effective antifungal, in addition to having anti-parasitic, antiviral and bactericidal properties. Research has shown that Olive Tree Extract contains almost double the antioxidant capacity than that of green tea.

As with many herbal treatments, Olive Leaf Extract has other, positive effects on your system. It contains antioxidant properties that are even more powerful than Vitamins C and E, Grape Seed Extract or Green Tea. This powerful antioxidant can help protect your body from aging and illness.

How does Olive Leaf Extract work?

Olive Leaf Extract stimulates your immune system's response to unwelcome invaders like Candida. It has also been shown to help stabilize blood sugar levels – this is important for sufferers because elevated blood sugar levels can feed your yeast overgrowth.

An added bonus for sufferers is that Olive Leaf Extract gives the body a natural energy boost. As anyone who has endured an infestation of Candidiasis knows, low energy levels are one of the primary symptoms of an outbreak.

How do I take Olive Leaf Extract?

Look for solutions with 20 percent *Oleuropein* if you can only find the 10 percent solution then just double the dosage.

Olive Leaf Extract Capsules (500mg)
Take 2 capsules 3 times daily with meals

Olive Leaf Extract Tea
Can be used once the symptoms are under control as a
preventative (maybe 1-3 cups a day).

Olive Leaf Extract Side Effects

Olive Leaf Extract is powerful enough to produce
uncomfortable Candida Die-Off symptoms quite quickly.
This means that it's important to take a smaller dose at first,
and be sure to drink lots of water.

Die-Off symptoms might cause some discomfort, but
remember that this is really good news – it means the
treatment is working.

Who should not take Olive Leaf Extract?

Those who should not take this product include women who
are pregnant or nursing, those who are diabetic or taking
medicine for high blood pressure, and finally anyone with
allergies to the pollen of the olive tree. If you have any
doubts, remember to consult your health professional.

Oregano Oil

Oregano is one of the most powerful antifungals, antiviral,
antibacterial and antiparasitic natural remedy, so oregano oil
is an excellent antifungal to start using for your treatment.
Oregano oil is particularly useful for treating an infestation.
One advantage that oregano oil has over other antifungals is
that the Candida yeast does not develop resistance, whereas
some other antifungals may lose effectiveness over time as
the yeast adapts to them. For the best results, take oregano oil

after you have finished your cleanse and use it in combination with one or two other natural antifungal.

How does Oregano Oil work?

Oregano oil contains two naturally occurring antimicrobial agents named *carvacrol* and *thymol*. Research suggests that these chemicals react with the water in your bloodstream to dehydrate and kill the yeast cells. Studies found that *carvacrol* was a more effective antimicrobial than 18 different pharmaceutical drugs. Oregano oil is entirely natural; it also tends to have fewer side effects than the regular antifungals that you might find in your pharmacy.

How should you take Oregano Oil?

If you buy oregano oil in a bottle, start by drinking 3 drops in water twice daily. You can gradually increase this up to 6 drops twice a day. It's best to drink one glass of water per 3 drops to prevent any burning in your mouth.

Also, you can buy oregano oil in a gel form. This is just as potent, and you can make it part of your daily vitamin and supplement routine. You can start with one soft gel, taken twice daily after meals, then work up to two soft gels twice a day.

Longer term, oregano can also be used to prevent a recurrence of your overgrowth. Oregano is an excellent supplement to take with many benefits for your health.

Who should not take Oregano Oil?

People with iron deficiencies should be aware that oregano oil can temporarily impair the body's ability to absorb iron. Pregnant women should avoid oregano oil as it could increase blood flow to the uterus weakening the lining surrounding the fetus.

Some patients may notice a small allergic reaction to the oil, in the form of rashes on the skin. Oregano Oil is essentially very safe though. If you have any doubts, contact your doctor.

Pau d'Arco

Pau d'Arco, is one of a number of herbal medicines that has come out of the Amazon rainforest in recent years. As doctors find antibiotics less and less effective against mutating diseases, they are looking to nature for answers and this is one of the more promising options

How does Pau d'Arco work?

Pau d'Arco's effects are dual when it comes to fungi. First the herb helps to loosen the bowels. Not enough to cause diarrhea, but enough to wash out old fecal matter and expose the yeast.

Secondly, Pau d'Arco acts as a powerful antifungal agent. It contains several classes of compounds, lapachol, xyloidone and various napthaquinones. The most important of these is lapachol, which has been shown to inhibit the growth.

How do you take Pau d'Arco?

Probably the easiest way to take Pau d'Arco is in tea. Teabags are available from many online pharmacies and supplement stores. This tea makes an excellent replacement for coffee and caffeinated beverages.

Who should not take Pau d'Arco?

Pregnant or breastfeeding women should not take Pau D'Arco. Also at risk are sufferers of blood thinning disorders, or those anticipating imminent surgery, as Pau D'Arco can thin the blood.

Pau d'Arco Side Effects

If used in large quantities Pau D'Arco has sometimes been found to weaken the immune system, so keep your doses small.

Candida Diet

Alternative practitioners recommend individualized programs that usually combine diet and supplements. Supplements are introduced gradually to avoid a temporary worsening of the symptoms called "die-off" or *Herxheimer reaction*. When the organisms are killed they release protein fragments and toxins that can trigger an antibody response from the immune system, it's because of this that it usually takes 2 to 3 weeks to see an improvement in symptoms. (We'll cover die-off symptoms and ways to manage them a little later in this guide).

Foods to Avoid on the Candida Cleanse

1. **Sugar-** Refined sugar is thought to encourage the growth of this yeast. Foods containing refined sugar include- white sugar, brown sugar, honey, maple syrup, corn syrup, maple sugar, molasses, date sugar, turbinado, raw sugar, demerrara, amasake, rice syrup and sorghum.

   Read label carefully because there may be hidden forms of sugar. When reading the label the words to watch out for include-sucrose, fructose, maltose, lactose, glycogen, glucose, mannitol, sorbitol, galactose, monosaccharide's and polysaccharide's.

2. **Fruit-** Fruit contains natural sugars that are thought to support the growth of yeast. Fruit that are typically eliminated include fresh fruit, frozen, canned, and dried fruit and fruit juice. Avoid raisins, bananas, raspberries and strawberries.

   Fruit Guidelines:

a. Avoid fruit which tastes too sweet Avoid fruit with mold on it

b. Avoid under-ripe and over-ripe fruit

c. Raw fruits have live enzymes and are quickly digested when eaten alone. Eaten with other foods, raw fruits take too long to digest and they stay too long in the digestive tract, where they become over-processed and a great food for this yeast to grow. The live enzymes in cooked fruits have been killed so the cooked fruit may be eaten with other foods and are digested like other carbohydrate foods. People with Candid have an easier time digesting cooked fruit than they do raw fruits.

3. **Yeast** - a diet containing yeasty foods such as white bread, pasta, dry breakfast cereals, pastry, potato chips, corn chips and white crackers seem to contribute to the growth.

4. **Cheeses**- all cheeses except ricotta, cottage cheese and cream cheeses. Use sparingly for some; the additives added to soft cheeses can aggravate the Candida and cause digestive problems.

5. **Artificially sweetened and sugary drinks and food products** should not be used. Avoid honey, maple syrup, fruit concentrate, fruit juice, sweet fruit and sugar, which can promote growth.

6. **Alcoholic Beverages**-these beverages are fermented-anything fermented contains yeasts.

7. Avoid all **fruit juices**, with the exception of fresh lemon or lime, which may be used in water or as a substitute for vinegar in salad dressings.

8. All **coffee and tea**, except for Pau de Arco and herbal teas.

9. **Chlorinated tap water**-this seems to be agreed upon by many researchers and suffers. Use pure, distilled water instead.

10. All **processed meats** including- bacon, sausage, ham, hot dogs, luncheon meats, corned beef and pastrami.

11. **Leftovers** which have been in the refrigerator for more than 3 days-don't eat them. Leftovers may be frozen and later thawed in the refrigerator, reheated and eaten immediately.

12. **Fungus foods**- all mushrooms, some say shiitake mushrooms are okay, but for the Candida diet to be effective, avoid all mushrooms, whether cooked or not cooked.

13. **Peanuts** and peanut products such as peanut butters. Use almond butter instead.

14. Basically when you first start the cleanse avoid **anything which has undergone a fermentation process** such as, soy sauce, miso, tamari, etc. Some people can tolerate small amounts others need to avoid it completely.

15. All **vinegar soaked products or vinegar dressings**- this includes white vinegar, red wine vinegar, rice vinegar, and balsamic vinegar. Avoid any foods made with vinegar such as mayonnaise, commercial salad dressings, ketchup, Worcestershire sauce, steak sauce, BBQ sauce, soy sauce, mustard, pickles, pickle relish,

sweet pickles, pickled vegetables, green olives, horseradish and chili sauce. For some people raw, unfiltered apple cider vinegar is tolerated and can be used without difficulty. Lemon and lime juice may be substituted for vinegar in recipes.

16. **Brewer's yeast, B Vitamins** which contain yeast.

What Can You Eat on the Candida Diet?

The above may seem like many tasty options are eliminated from the Candida Diet, yet the variety of foods allowed on the diet are delicious and non-yeast producing. You won't miss the over-processed and high sugar foods you ate before. Take a look at the wonderful variety available to you!

1. **Meats**- Chicken, turkey, all game birds, quail, duck, goose, pheasant, and Cornish hens. Grass-fed beef, buffalo, lamb, and venison. The meat you purchase must be antibiotic and hormone free.

2. **Eggs**- Choose Omega-3 free range fertilized eggs in moderation. The eggs should be well cooked to be considered safe during the treatment. Avoid soft-boiled, sunny-side up or quick cooked eggs-totally avoid raw eggs. One or two servings per week is fine for most people, unless they are allergic to eggs.

3. **Fish**-All fresh fish including salmon, cod, herring, sardines, shrimp, lobster and oysters. Wild is best.

4. **Nuts, seeds and unprocessed oils**, almonds, brazil nuts, cashews, filberts, pecans, pumpkin seeds, sunflower seeds and sesame seeds. Avoid roasted and salted nuts and seeds.

5. **Cold pressed oils**- almond, avocado, flax seed, butter, apricot, corn, walnut, sunflower, olive and sesame oil. Be careful that they are not rancid; add two capsules of vitamin E per cup of stored oil to prevent it from turning rancid.

6. **Whole grains**-including quinoa, amaranth, buckwheat, rye, (after the first 2 weeks, try whole wheat and oats.)

7. **Crackers and chips**-any whole grain, unsweetened crackers or chips made with the above grains, including Koyo brand buckwheat rice cakes, Rye Vita brand crackers in various flavors.

8. **Muffins & Biscuits**: Any whole grain muffin, biscuit, tortilla, - must be made with soda or baking powder - not yeast. Use approved flours.

9. **Legumes**: All legumes such as lentils, peas, soybeans, pinto, navy, northern, kidney etc.

10. **Fresh Vegetables**: All vegetables (be adventurous) including asparagus, beets broccoli, cabbage, carrots, cauliflower, celery, cucumbers, eggplant, green peppers, greens, lettuce, turnip, spinach, onions, peas, parsley, fresh tomatoes, squash (summer, winter, butter, zucchini), red potatoes (no white), radishes, okra, parsnip, collards, yams and avocados.

11. **Extras for Taste**: Lemons and limes are great to spruce up a salad or other recipes – (After 1st 2 weeks may use miso and soy sauce) Use stevia, xylitol and erithritol as natural sweeteners

12. **Dairy**: Avoid dairy for the first 2 weeks. May use unsweetened yogurt with approved berries or xylitol,

goat milk and soft goat cheese. Use unsweetened Almond milk or Hemp milk.

13. **Beverages**: Bottled, filtered water and sparkling water with lemons or limes. Hot or room temperatures.

Healing Drinks for the Cleanse

Detox Drink

- 1 cup of water

- 1 teaspoon Psylluim Husk powder

- 1 teaspoon Bentonite Clay

Psylluim and Bentonite clay don't mix very well with water, so shake the mixture well for a few seconds then drink quickly. Drink another large glass of water immediately after.

This may not sound like an appetizing drink but Psylluim and Bentonite clay are great for detox. The Bentonite clay soaks up the toxins and Psylluim pushes the waste material out through your colon.

Liver Flush Drink

- 1 cup water

- 1 tablespoon extra virgin olive oil

- 1 clove garlic

- Small chunk of ginger root

Using a blender, blend all ingredients together and drink in the evening 2 hours after last detox drink.

Remember drink plenty of water during the day to assist with the toxin flush process.

Breakfast Recipes

Warming Buckwheat Cereal

If you're looking for simple breakfast recipes to use while on your diet, this is a great option. The combination of buckwheat and oat bran makes for a tasty, filling porridge. After the first week you can start to reintroduce foods such as some chopped green apple for some extra flavor.

Ingredients

- 1/4 cup buckwheat groats
- 1/4 cup oat bran
- 1/2 cup coconut milk
- 2 Tbsp. coconut oil
- Cinnamon
- Stevia to taste

Preparation

Cook the buckwheat groats and oat bran as directed. You may need to start the buckwheat first and then add the oat bran, depending on the recommended cooking time for each one.

Drain the water, and then stir in the coconut oil and coconut milk.

Mix in cinnamon and add some Stevia to taste.

Veggie Omelet

Eating eggs is a great way to give you energy for the rest of the morning. This simple omelet recipe is healthy, delicious and satisfying, and it's perfect for this diet. You can also use coconut oil instead of the olive oil if you prefer. Limit the amount of eggs to 2 during the first week of the cleanse- after the first week you may consume no more than 6 organic eggs, per week.

Ingredients

- 2-3 organic eggs
- 2 Tbsp. olive oil
- 1/2 small onion, chopped
- 1/2 red pepper, chopped
- Handful of fresh spinach
- Sea salt

Preparation

Heat a skillet with the olive oil.

Start cooking the onions and peppers, then add the spinach a few minutes later.

Stir fry until veggies are tender.

Now stir in the slightly beaten eggs until eggs are done.

Season with sea salt and serve.

Lunch & Dinner Recipes

Chicken and Quinoa

This recipe is great for a low-sugar diet like the treatment plan. It's a simple recipe with lean protein and lots of vegetables, and it uses a dressing of lemon, olive oil and salt.

Ingredients

- 1 chicken breast

- 2/3 cup of cooked quinoa
- 2 cups of spinach
- 2 medium tomatoes
- 1/2 cucumber
- 1 avocado
- 2 shallots
- 1 garlic clove, minced
- Juice of 1/2 lemon
- 2 Tbsp. olive oil
- Sea salt

Preparation

Cook the quinoa as directed.

Chop up the chicken and pan-fry with the minced garlic until cooked thoroughly (about 5 minutes).

Now chop up the veggies, toss everything in a bowl and serve. Delicious!

Soba Noodle Veggie Bowl

This Asian-inspired dish is really simple to prepare, filling and very tasty. Soba noodles are made from buckwheat groats. They have a lower glycemic index than regular noodles and a great alternative if you're on the diet.

Ingredients

- 2 oz. soba noodles

- 1/4 cup dry Wakame seaweed
- 2 tomatoes
- 1 avocado
- 2 Tbsp. sesame oil
- Sprinkle of sesame seeds
- Salt to taste

Preparation

Soak the seaweed in a bowl with warm water for about 10 minutes.

Boil the soba noodles for 6 minutes.

Chop the tomatoes and avocado then add everything to a bowl and mix.

Drizzle with sesame oil and sprinkle with the sesame seeds. Serves 2.

Snack Recipes

Muhammara

Muhammara is a tasty dish that originates in Syria. It is usually sweetened with pomegranate molasses, but this version has no added sugar or sweeteners and is great for the diet plan.

Ingredients

- 3 red peppers
- 1 small red onion
- 3/4 cup walnuts

- 1-2 garlic cloves
- 1/4 cup olive oil
- 1/4 tsp. cayenne pepper
- 1/4 tsp. cumin
- Juice of 1/2 lemon
- Salt to taste

Preparation

Roast the peppers for 10-12 minutes at 350 degrees F on a greased baking tray, turning approximately every 4 minutes.

When finished, peel off the skin from the peppers and remove the seeds and stem.

Chop and saute the onions for 3-5 minutes.

Now add all ingredients to the food processor.

Serve with quinoa crackers or sliced vegetables for dipping.

Herbed Flat Bread

Bread is one of the items that can cause problems for those of us who have a problem with yeast. This bread won't feed it- instead it is a preventative, due to the ingredients. This bread is so yummy with the Muhammara dip.

Ingredients

- 2 Tbsp. olive oil
- 1 leek, sliced into thin rings
- 3 cloves roasted garlic, mashed
- 4 egg whites
- 4 egg yolks

- 1/3 cup kefir
- 1/3 cup coconut flour, sifted
- 1/3 cup golden flaxseed meal
- 1/2 teaspoon salt
- 1/4 tsp. baking soda
- 1 tsp. Herbs de Provence
- Salt and pepper to taste

Directions

Heat 1 tablespoon of olive oil in a skillet over medium low heat. Add sliced leek and sauté until softened, but not browned, about 5 minutes. Remove from heat and mix in mashed roasted garlic cloves, set aside.

Preheat oven to 350 degrees F (175 degrees C). With a brush, oil a 13×9 inch baking pan with olive oil. Cut a piece of parchment paper the width of the bottom of the baking pan and long enough to overlap the ends of the pan. Brush parchment paper with olive oil, set aside.

In a medium bowl, beat egg whites until soft peaks form, set aside. In a small bowl, whisk egg yolks and kefir, set aside. In a large bowl, combine sifted coconut flour, golden flaxseed meal, salt and baking soda. Fold egg whites and egg yolk mixture into flour mixture until just combined.

Spread batter evenly in prepared baking pan and bake for 10 minutes. Remove baking pan from oven and scatter top of bread with leek and roasted garlic mixture, drizzle with remaining 1 tablespoon of olive oil, season with Herbs de Provence and salt and pepper to taste. Return baking pan to oven and bake bread for another 10 minutes, or until edges begin to brown.

Cool, slice, serve. It also makes great bread for sandwiches! Delicious with a veggie dip.

Roasted Garlic

Preheat oven to 400 degrees F (200 degrees C). Slice off top quarter of a whole head of garlic. Place garlic head in a small baking dish, cut side up, and drizzle with 1 tablespoon of olive oil. Cover baking dish tightly with foil and bake for 1 hour. Let garlic cool slightly before using. Refrigerate unused portion in an airtight container for 1 to 2 weeks.

Dessert Recipes

Coconut Ginger Cookies

Yes, you can have sweets, and these cookies won't cause a rise in your blood sugar!

These coconut ginger cookies contain three different types of coconut – coconut milk, coconut oil and coconut flour. All three are low in sugars and have antifungal properties. I also like to add some grated ginger to these cookies, just to give the flavor a little boost. This is a great snack to put in your bag and take out with you when you leave the house. Enjoy!

Ingredients

- 1 cup coconut flour
- 1/4 cup hemp seeds
- 1/4 tsp. salt
- 2 tsp. Stevia
- 1 can coconut milk (14oz / 400ml)

- 1/4 cup coconut oil, melted
- 4 eggs
- 2 Tbsp. fresh ginger, grated

Preparation

Preheat the oven to 350F. Place a piece of parchment paper on a baking sheet.

Add all the dry ingredients to the food processor (coconut flour, hemp seeds, stevia, and salt. Mix together add the rest of the ingredients. Pulse until it reaches an even consistency.

Use a tablespoon to drop the cookie dough on the baking sheet. Use your hand to shape each cookie as they won't spread on their own.

Bake for 12-14 minutes, until edges are brown.

Almond and Coconut Balls

Here is a delicious recipe that uses unsweetened almond butter and stevia. This recipe requires no baking at all. You can eat these no-bake balls in moderation during your diet.

Ingredients

- 1 cup almond butter (unsweetened)
- 1/2 cup coconut flour
- 1/2 cup unsweetened shredded coconut
- 4 Tbsp. coconut milk
- 4 Tbsp. coconut oil
- 1 packet of stevia

Preparation

Set aside a heaped tablespoon of the shredded coconut in a bowl.

Add all the other ingredients to a food processor and blend until nicely mixed together.

Now mold the mixture with your hands into bite sized balls, and roll them in the shredded coconut.

Place them on a plate and refrigerate for 30 minutes. Enjoy!

Beverages

Ginger Tea

This is one of my favorites. It's great for improving digestion supports your immune system, and you can drink it as much as you like during your diet. Great substitute for coffee!

- 1 square inch piece of fresh Ginger root
- Squeeze of lemon
- 2 cup of water

Cut off and discard the outside of the ginger root. Now grate the rest of the root and add to boiling water. Boil for 20 minutes. Strain and serve with a slice of lemon.

Smoothies are great for cleansing because they require little energy to be used by your digestive system, allowing the body to focus on rebuilding, renewing and healing. Here is a great one to try! Don't let the avocado scare you away this is truly yummy!

Avocado Cream Smoothie

- 1 medium avocado, peeled and pitted
- 1 cup coconut milk
- Stevia
- 6 ice cubes

Blend the avocado, Stevia, coconut milk, and ice together until smooth.

The 7-Day Colon Cleanse

This is an important part of the Candida Cleanse- this is the beginning of your battle to rid your body of the Candida overgrowth. By doing a 7 day colon cleanse you attack the very area where Candida has taken up residence and is growing and multiplying in sugary yeasty warmth. Instead we want to give these toxins big pushes out of our system with the help of the 21 day detox.

To begin, you start with a colonic on the first day, then on alternating days for the rest of the week. The colonic irrigation is an important part of this cleanse to completely eliminate the yeast and its toxins.

A simple colon cleanses usually lasts 1-2 weeks. After this, you can start taking the probiotics and antifungals.

As you begin your cleanse, you may start to experience some symptoms of Candida die-off. If you decide to try the colonics, the benefits of the irrigations are-as the yeast are killed and flushed out of the system, the colonics help to lessen the Candida die-off symptoms.

What is a Colonic?

A colonic session usually lasts about 45 minutes. For good results you should get a colonic every other day for a week. During the colonic you will be asked to lie down and is given a gentle but firm massage to the lower stomach area. The reason for the massage is to loosen up the waste matter that the colonic will flush out.

Then a small sterile and disposable plastic tube is then inserted into the rectum and warm water is passed into the colon. Most people experience a warm feeling but do not usually report much sensation or discomfort. For some do say they feel slightly uncomfortable at first, then it subsides.

The water is then allowed to gently flow into your colon, and you push it out along with the fecal matter that has been loosened. This cycle is repeated several times. Occasionally other liquids-such as coffee is added to the water, to help with further loosening of the matter. Colonics rid the colon of the overgrowth and other toxins, which then will increase the healing effect of the cleanse and lessen the symptoms of the Candida die-off.

The Keys to a Successful Cleanse

- Eat raw organic salads and steamed vegetables

- Do the cleanse for at least 7-21 days-stop after 7 if your physician makes this recommendation

- Drink plenty of water to stay hydrated and to flush away the toxins

- Drink a detox drink (recipe) 3 times each day-morning, afternoon and evening

- Drink the liver flush (recipe) every evening at least 2 hours after your last detox drink

- Have a colonic irrigation every second day for 7 days (optional, but recommended)

- Continue the Cleansing Drinks up to the 21 days, and then begin the diet, slowly adding foods to the diet.

Candida Die-Off

During the cleanse some people may experience Candida die-off symptoms as they increase their intake of the supplements because the yeast has nothing to feed on anymore. To begin with you may feel worse before you feel better, but do not be worried or put off by an increase in symptoms because it means that your body is getting rid of all the toxins that have been causing the problem. These symptoms, if they occur, will usually occur in the second week.

Die-off symptoms:

a. Headaches
b. Nausea
c. Brain fog
d. Forgetfulness
e. Dizziness
f. Fatigue
g. Sugar cravings
h. Minor skin breakouts
i. Cold hands and feet
j. Diarrhea
k. Constipation
l. Bloating
m. May bruise easily
n. Lower resistance to colds, viruses, bacterial infections
o. Increase in mucus build-up

A person experiencing these symptoms is usually quite toxic. These symptoms are temporary and can last from a couple of days up to two weeks. If they persist, stop and see your health care provider.

Acupuncture can help lessen these symptoms. ***DO NOT*** discontinue your diet because of detoxification symptoms. You may question why you are on such a diet if it makes you feel so sick, but you are actually getting better. You will want to eat a diet that starves the yeast, keeps an acid/alkaline balance: The human body should normally be slightly alkaline. However, many experts feel that the Standard American diet contributes to our acidic state.

How to Cope with Candida Die-off

Die-off can be difficult for some people, especially if they have a serious case of overgrowth. There are ways to make the die-off easier to cope with your physician's permission. If the symptoms become severe, notify your doctor immediately.

Candidate- Is a 100% herbal solution that can support you during the die-off by helping your liver remove toxins more quickly from your body.

Molybdenum- Converts acetaldehyde (the major toxin released during die-off) into acetic acid. This can then be excreted from the body like any other toxin.

Vitamin C- Restores your adrenal function and helps to boost your immune system.

Milk Thistle-This herb contains a compound that helps to repair damaged liver cells and protect them from the toxins released in die-off.

Swedish Bitters- Are an excellent digestive support. They also help to regulate your stomach acidity and support your liver function.

Detox Drops- Is a supplement that promotes the healthy functioning of your liver and the elimination of toxins from your body.

Alternative Detox Methods

These alternative methods often help assist with the detox process, not only do they help to remove toxins from the system, but it feels like pampering and soothing to your taxed body.

Oil Pulling- This ancient remedy mystifies modern doctors, but anecdotal evidence suggests it can help reduce the symptoms of die-off. Oil pulling originated in Ayurvedic literature. It is a safe simple treatment which anyone can do. You simply swish oil around in your mouth, then spit it out. Oil pulling eliminates the yeast from oral thrush and expels the toxins. Oil pulling can be used at any stage of your treatment. Many Naturopaths recommend it as a part of your daily morning routine.

Oil pulling is an easy process, but there are some rules you must follow.

1. After brushing your teeth in the morning, put one tablespoon of extra virgin coconut oil in your mouth, then swish it around like mouthwash.
2. Make sure you swish it all over your mouth, between the teeth, under the tongue, across the roof of your mouth.
3. Do this for 15 minutes if you can.
4. Now spit it out and rinse your mouth with salt water.

Rules to remember:

1. Do oil pulling on an empty stomach
2. Don't swallow the oil! By the time you finish swishing it is full of pathogens and toxins.
3. Remember spit it out.
4. Don't gargle with the oil.

Skin Brushing-Your skin is responsible for up to 15% of toxin elimination. Skin brushing enhances this process and improves your circulation too.

Following these instructions will make skin brushing more effective.

1. Begin your skin brushing before you shower or bathe and use a dry brush.
2. Start on the soles of your feet using small circular motions.
3. Move to your legs using long strokes. Always brush towards your chest following the flow of the lymphatic fluid.
4. Go counter clockwise on your stomach and abdomen.
5. Move to your arms, starting at the fingertips and brush towards your body. Use small circular strokes in your armpits.
6. Then brush your shoulders and upper chest always towards your heart.
7. Take a shower and dry yourself thoroughly.
8. Avoid any broken or infected skin areas. If you wish to use an oil after your shower, use coconut oil, because it's a great antifungal.

Use a brush with natural, firm bristles. Don't use a brush with synthetic bristles because they can scratch the skin and may have toxic chemicals in the bristles. Wash your brush with soap and water every couple of weeks to remove dead skin cells. Each brush should last a few months before you need to replace it.

Contrast Showers- Boost your lymphatic system and improve your circulation. They have long been used as an alternative remedy for the common cold. Naturopaths believe contrast showers can improve your circulation and boost your immunity. Both will help to fight your Candida overgrowth.

How to take a Contrast Shower:

1. Shower in warm/hot water (not scalding) for 3-5 minutes
2. Now turn off the hot water and shower under cool/cold water for 1 minute **only.**
3. Repeat 3-5 times.
4. Make sure to finish with cold water.

Note: If you have heart disease, high blood pressure, asthma or diabetes, you should consult with your physician before trying contrast showers and pregnant women should avoid this therapy altogether.

Exercise and Candida-The right amount of exercise can improve your body's defenses against Candida. Walking, jogging, biking, yoga, etc are excellent choices. Don't over-do it though as this can weaken your adrenals.

Sauna- Improves circulation and helps you flush out toxins through sweating.

Candida Reoccurrence and Beyond

You have followed the Candida Cleanse, changed your diet, and gave up coffee and sugar, yet the yeast returns, just when you think you are cured.

Or...

Sometimes people who have cleared their systems of yeast are feeling so great, they may actually slip and eat something which they have an allergy to (an allergic reaction such as a rash- can actually be due Candida) or which sparks a new overgrowth.

To remain healthy and free of yeast infections continue taking the supplements, probiotics and antifungals, unless your physician advises otherwise. Avoid the foods which cause an outbreak, you will know if a food is to be avoided, due to the return of the symptoms.

Guidelines for a Lifetime of Candida Control

1. Do not eat sweets on an empty stomach. Have a meal first or a protein snack.

2. Eat dessert 1 to 1 ½ hours after having a full meal.

3. Take a vitamin B complex once or twice each day and at least 500 mg vitamin C daily.

4. If you are drinking alcohol, limit the drinks to two drinks maximum and make sure you don't have an empty stomach and avoid sweet wines and alcoholic drinks.

5. Avoid drinking alcohol more than 2 to 8 days per month.

6. Drink tested, filtered spring water, don't drink chlorinated tap water.

7. Do a vegetable fast occasionally as needed, one to four times per month. It will rest your digestive system and purge body toxins.

8. Keep a food diary and watch for reactions to certain foods or combinations of foods. Inform your physician of the results.

Now that you have been free of the Candida overgrowth, keep the yeasties at bay, take care of yourself and enjoy your life.

Conclusion

Thank you again for purchasing this book!

I hope it was valuable to you not only as a Candida sufferer, but also to help to prevent Candida overgrowths in the first place.

The next step is to educate yourself by reading more material concerning Candida. Understanding and knowledge are the best medicine!

Finally, if you enjoyed this book, please take the time to share your thoughts and post a review on Amazon. It'd be greatly appreciated!

Thank you and good luck!

Christine Weil

Check out the other books in the *Natural Health & Natural Cures Series*

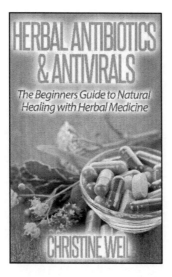

https://www.amazon.com/dp/B00J2F1QDO

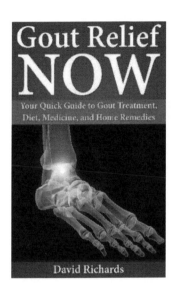

http://www.amazon.com/dp/B00HHGRBBQ

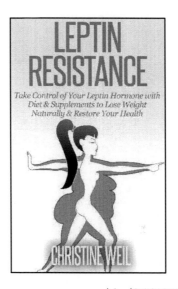

http://www.amazon.com/dp/B00J8UNBWW

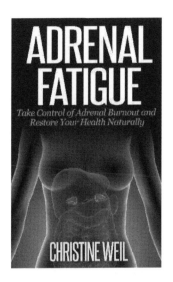

http://www.amazon.com/dp/B00J8SHS6E

Made in the USA
San Bernardino, CA
28 September 2014